Brain Fuel: Empower and Increase Brain Function with These Delicious Dishes

All rights Reserved. No part of this publication or the information in it may be quoted from or reproduced in any form by means such as printing, scanning, photocopying or otherwise without prior written permission of the copyright holder.

Disclaimer and Terms of Use: Effort has been made to ensure that the information in this book is accurate and complete, however, the author and the publisher do not warrant the accuracy of the information, text and graphics contained within the book due to the rapidly changing nature of science, research, known and unknown facts and Internet. The Author and the publisher do not hold any responsibility for errors, omissions or contrary interpretation of the subject matter herein. This book is presented solely for motivational and informational purposes only.

Table of Contents

Smoothies

Serves: 2
Cooking Time: 5 minutes

Ingredients

2/3 cup Greek yogurt
1 banana
2/3 cup blueberries, frozen
2 large strawberries
1 cup spinach
1/2 cup almond milk
2 tsp protein powder
1 tbsp honey

Directions

I.   Add everything into a blender or food processor.
II.   Blend until smooth.

Nutritional Information

Calories 202, Fat 1.2g, Protein 4.4g, Carbs 47g, Fiber 5.5g

Serves: 2
Cooking Time: 5 minutes

Ingredients

1 kiwi, peeled and chopped
½ avocado, peeled and chopped
1 cup baby spinach
1 cup apple juice

Directions

I. Add everything into a blender or food processor.
II. Blend until smooth.

Nutritional Information

Calories 81, Fat 3.5g, Protein .9g, Carbs 12.8g, Fiber 2.4g

Fruit Spinach Smoothie

Serves: 2
Cooking Time: 5 minutes

Ingredients

½ cup water
1 cup spinach
½ bag mixed fruit, frozen

Directions

I.   Add everything into a blender or food processor.
II.   Blend until smooth.

Nutritional Information

Calories 81.7, Fat 3.5g, Protein .9g, 12.8g, Fiber 2.4g

Berry Spinach Smoothie

Serves: 2
Cooking Time: 5 minutes

Ingredients

1 cup baby spinach, frozen
1 ½ cups blueberries, frozen
½ cup raspberries, frozen
1 cup orange juice

Directions

I.   Add everything into a blender or food processor.
II.   Blend until smooth.

Nutritional Information

Calories 87, Fat .8g, Carbs 20g, Protein 31g

Serves: 2
Cooking Time: 5 minutes

Ingredients

> 4 cups baby spinach, fresh
> 6 oz plain yogurt
> 1 banana
> ½ cup water

Directions

> I.   Add everything into a blender or food processor.
> II. Blend until smooth.

Nutritional Information

> Calories 77, Fat 18g, Carbs 20g, Protein 31g

Serves: 2
Cooking Time: 5 minutes

Ingredients

2 cups baby spinach
½ cup coconut milk
½ cup ice
½ granny smith apple
1 lime, juiced

Directions

I.   Add all of the ingredients into a blender or food
        processor.
II.   Blend on high until smooth.

Nutritional Information

Calories 81, Fat 3.5g, Protein .9g, Carbs 12.8g

Morning

Serves: 1
Cooking Time: 15 minutes

Ingredients

1 egg
1 tsp olive oil
1 English muffin
1 slice Swiss cheese
1 slice tomato
2 to 3 spinach leaves

Directions

I.   Fry an egg in the olive oil.
II.   Slice the English muffin in half (toast if you desire).
III.   Layer with the egg and remaining ingredients.

Nutritional Information

Calories 360, Fat 12g, Carbs 50g, Protein 20g

Serves: 1
Cooking Time: 8 to 12 minutes

Ingredients

2 whole grain waffles
½ cup frozen berries (thawed)
½ cup plain yogurt
2 tsp ground flaxseed

Directions

I.   Garnish the waffles with the yogurt and berries.
II.   Sprinkle flaxseed over top.

Nutritional Information

Calories 367, Fat 11.5g, Carbs 44g, Protein 24g

Serves: 1
Cooking Time: 10 to 15 minutes

Ingredients

¼ cup canned pumpkin spread
1 pear, chopped
1 tsp honey
¾ cup plain yogurt
½ cup Kashi cereal
1 tbsp walnuts, chopped

Directions

I.   Spread pumpkin, ½ of the pear and honey into the yogurt.
II.   Stir in the remaining ingredients.

Nutritional Information

Calories 362, Fat 2.5g, Carbs 61g, Protein 19g

Serves: 1
Cooking Time: 1 to 2 minutes

Ingredients

   2 slices whole wheat bread
   ¼ cup cottage cheese
   2 slices red onion
   2 oz smoked salmon
   1 glass orange juice

Directions

   I.   Toast your bread in a toaster.
   II.   Spread cottage cheese over toast, garnish with salmon
           and onion.
   III.   Enjoy with a cold glass of orange juice.

Nutritional Information

   Calories 338, Fat 4.5g, Carbs 52g, Protein 24g

Serves: 1
Cooking Time: 4 to 5 minutes

Ingredients

½ cup oats
2 tbsp raisins
¼ cup apple, chopped
1 tbsp almonds, slivered
4 to 6 oz plain yogurt
2 oz 2% milk
1 tsp brown sugar to garnish

Directions

Combine everything together, toss.

Nutritional Information

Calories 361, Fat 2g, Carbs 57g, Protein 17g

Serves: 1
Cooking Time: 10 to 12 minutes

Ingredients

¾ cup whole grain cereal
½ cup high fiber cereal of your choice
4 tsp pumpkin seeds
1 peach, sliced and pitted
8 oz almond milk

Directions

I.   Combine both dry cereals together and toss in container with a lid.
II.   Add in the pumpkin seeds and toss a little more.
III.   Pour into cereal bowl and add milk.
IV.   Top with peach to garnish.

Nutritional Information

Calories 348, Fat 1g, Carbs 75g, Protein 318g

Anytime

Serves: 2
Cooking Time: 15 to 20 minutes

Ingredients

1 tbsp EVOO
1 sweet onion, sliced
1 cup baby spinach
salt & pepper to taste
1 pear, cored and sliced
1 oz blue cheese, crumbled

Directions

I.   Add olive oil to a skillet and heat, sauté the onions until they are caramelized. This should take 10 to 15 minutes; once they are heated, set aside.
II. Wash and dry the spinach, chop and add to the warm skillet for just 1 to 2 minutes, season with salt and pepper to taste.
III. Add remaining ingredients and toss together.

Nutritional Information

Calories 81, Fat 3.5g, Protein .9g, Carbs 12.8g

Warm Spinach & Beets

Serves: 2
Cooking Time: 40 minutes

Ingredients

- 8 cups baby spinach
- 1 tbsp EVOO
- 1 cup red onions, sliced
- 2 tomatoes, chopped
- 2 tbsp olives
- 2 tbsp parsley, chopped
- 1 tbsp garlic, minced
- 2 cup beets, steamed and chopped
- 2 tbsp balsamic vinegar
- ¼ tsp salt and pepper to taste

Directions

I.   Add the spinach to a large bowl.
II.   In a skillet heat, heat the oil and add the onion, stir and wait until the onion softens.
III.   Add in the tomatoes, olives and remaining ingredients, cook for about 2 to 3 minutes.
IV.   Add the blend to the spinach and toss well.
V.   Serve warm

Nutritional Information

Calories 81, Fat 3.5g, Protein .9g, Carbs 12.8g

Serves: 1
Cooking Time: 15 to 20 minutes

Ingredients

3 tbsp olive oil
2 tbsp garlic, minced
lemon juice
¼ tsp salt and pepper
5 4 to 6 oz baby spinach
1 lb cooked orzo
1 c pitted olives, pitted
4 oz feta cheese, crumbled
¼ c red onions, sliced
¼ c mint leaves, chopped

Directions

I.   Heat oil and sauté garlic, salt and pepper in a saucepan.
II.   Add remaining ingredients and cook for 1 to 2 minutes.
III.   Toss lightly and serve.

Nutritional Information

Calories 361, Fat 13g, Carbs 48g, Protein 31g

Serves: 1
Cooking Time: 15 minutes

Ingredients

¾ cup yogurt
½ cup shredded wheat
¼ cup fiber cereal
1 tbsp walnuts, chopped
¼ banana, sliced
¼ cup mixed berries

Directions

Layer the ingredients in a parfait cup in the order they are listed.

Nutritional Information

Calories 336, Fat 16g, Carbs 10g, Protein 59g

Serves: 6 to 8
Cooking Time: 30 to 45 minutes

Ingredients

4 cups pinto beans, dry
2 tbsp EVOO
1 onion, chopped
3 tbsp garlic, minced
1 carrot, shaved
2 ½ cup kale, chopped
1 cup tomato sauce
3 tbsp chili powder
1 tbsp oregano
1 tsp cinnamon
1 tsp cocoa powder, dark chocolate
1 can chipotle pepper in adobo sauce (reserve and save 1 tbsp sauce)
salt and pepper

Directions

I.   Rinse the beans, add them to a large stock pot for 8 hours. Let the beans soak overnight.

II.   When you are ready to cook, add oil to a pan and then add the garlic, onion, carrot and kale. Sauté for 2 to 4 minutes.

III.   Transfer food from skillet to the pot with the beans.

IV.   Add remaining ingredients to the stock pot and bring everything to a boil. Cook for about an hour but check it often to make sure the beans don't dry out. Add water as needed.

V.   When everything is ready, serve or freeze.

Nutritional Information

Calories 377, Fat 18g, Carbs 20g, Protein 31g

Serves: 2
Cooking Time: 2 to 4 minutes

Ingredients

1/3 cup raw almonds
1 tsp honey
1 tbsp cocoa powder, dark
1 banana
1 cup ice

Directions

I.   Soak the almonds for around 6 to 8 hours or overnight, if possible.
II.   Drain water from the almonds and add them to your blender or food processor.
III.   Add 1 cup water and remaining ingredients.
IV.   Blend until smooth.

Nutritional Information

Calories 377, Fat 18g, Carbs 20g, Protein 31g

Serves: 20
Cooking Time: 30 to 45 minutes

Ingredients

½ cup + 2 tbsp flour
5 tbsp flaxseed, ground
6 tbsp powdered sugar
½ tsp powdered cardamom
½ cup soft butter
1 tbsp sour cream
3 tbsp marmalade

Directions

I.   Sift the dry ingredients together and stir in the butter and sour cream.
II.   Form small balls from the dough and place on a baking sheet covered in parchment paper.
III.   Preheat oven to 350 °F.
IV.   Divide the dough balls in half and using your thumb, make a small, pressed indention in the center of the dough balls.
V.   Bake for 12 to 15 minutes.
VI.   Let them cool, then add a small spoonful of marmalade into the indention.

Nutritional Information

Calories 377, Fat 18g, Carbs 20g, Protein 31g

Serves: 4
Cooking Time: 25 to 45 minutes

Ingredients

4 artichokes, trimmed
7 tbsp olive oil
1 onion, chopped
2 tbsp garlic, minced
1 ¼ cup bread crumbs
2 oz chili peppers, roasted and minced

Gremolata
¼ cup parsley, chopped
1 tbsp minced garlic, minced
1 tsp lemon zest

Yogurt Sauce

½ cup Greek yogurt
1 tbsp garlic, minced
1 tsp lemon zest

Directions

I. Fill a large saucepan with water and add artichoke pieces to water and bring to a boil for about 30 to 45 minutes. Remove and set them upside down to drain and cool.

II. In a skillet, add 2 tbsp oil and sauté the onion and garlic. Add it to a bowl with the bread crumbs, parmesan cheese, salt and pepper, and toss.

III. Add the rest of the oil and stir well.

IV. Remove soft or fuzzy part of the artichokes and hollow out so that you can stuff artichokes with the bread mixture. Let set in fridge overnight.

V.   Make your Gremolata by combining all of the ingredients and stirring well.
VI.   For the yogurt sauce, blend the ingredients together and cool until ready to use.
VII.   Preheat broiler, add artichokes to a baking sheet and top with the rest of parmesan cheese or about ¼ cup. Broil until the cheese melts.
VIII.   Garnish artichokes with the Gremolata and Yogurt Sauce.

Nutritional Information

Calories 377, Fat 18g, Carbs 20g, Protein 31g

Serves: 16
Cooking Time: 1 hour and 30 minutes

Ingredients

1 lb almonds
1 egg white
1 tsp vanilla extract
¾ cup brown sugar
¼ cup sugar
½ tsp salt
2 tsp cinnamon

Directions

I.   Preheat oven to 225 °F.
II.   Whisk the egg white with vanilla until fluffy.
III.   Stir the almonds into the egg mix.
IV.   Add the remaining ingredients to a second bowl.
V.   Add the almonds into the sugar blend and toss to coat well.
VI.   Spread coated almonds out over baking dish and bake for an hour and 15 minutes.
VII.   Let cool.

Nutritional Information

Calories 377, Fat 18g, Carbs 20g, Protein 31g

Serves: 8 to 10
Cooking Time: 1 hour

Ingredients

- 1 cup strawberries, chopped
- 3 kiwis, chopped
- ¼ cup mango, chopped
- ½ cup pineapple, chopped
- 1 orange, peeled and chopped
- ¼ cup bell pepper, chopped
- ¼ cup green onion, sliced
- 1 tbsp lemon juice
- 1 jalapeño, chopped and seeded

Directions

I. Combine the fruits, peppers and other chopped ingredients in a bowl and toss.
II. Add plastic wrap over the bowl and let chill in fridge for 30 to 45 minutes.

Nutritional Information

Calories 377, Fat 18g, Carbs 20g, Protein 31g

www.ingramcontent.com/pod-product-compliance
Lightning Source LLC
Chambersburg PA
CBHW060351290526
45791CB00004B/1623